TRE FOR HEALING

Unlocking Trauma Release Exercises For Emotional Resilience, Stress Reduction, And Holistic Recovery

DR. MELISSA STOTLER

Disclaimer:

The data in this book, is solely meant to be informative and instructional.

This book is not intended to replace expert medical advice, diagnosis, or care. No medical, health, or other professional services are offered by the author, publisher, or any affiliated parties

Individual outcomes may differ in the practice of these therapies, which entail a variety of approaches and methodologies.

A one-on-one session with a trained or certified healthcare professional is still preferable. It is best to consult a trained healthcare provider before making any decisions regarding your health.

The author of this book is not affiliated with any specific website, product, or organization related to any of these therapies.

All reasonable measures have been taken by the author and publisher to guarantee the authenticity and dependability of the material contained in this book.

Contents

TRE (Tension and Trauma Releasing Exercises) represents a profound and innovative approach to healing, both physically and mentally. This book is a vital resource for anyone seeking to understand and harness the transformative power of TRE. It begins with a comprehensive introduction, detailing the origins and foundational principles of TRE, as well as its numerous benefits. Readers will learn how TRE supports mental and physical health, dispelling common misconceptions while providing practical guidance on getting started with this method.

The exploration of TRE's underlying science reveals how it interacts with the nervous system, emphasizing the role of tremors in facilitating healing. Neurogenic tremors are explained, illustrating their crucial impact on stress reduction and overall wellness. Through a review of recent research findings, readers gain insight into the effectiveness of TRE and its scientific backing.

Safety considerations are paramount in any healing practice, and this book addresses who should practice TRE, potential risks, and how to determine if it is appropriate for you. It offers essential safety guidelines and best practices, including advice on what to do if discomfort arises.

Preparation for TRE is covered in detail, guiding readers in setting up their practice space, choosing appropriate equipment and attire, and mentally preparing for the exercises. Emphasis is placed on creating a conducive environment and setting realistic goals to ensure a successful practice.

The core of the book focuses on the TRE practice itself, providing detailed instructions on basic exercises, integrating breathing techniques, and tailoring the practice to individual needs. Guidance on session duration, frequency, and common adjustments helps readers achieve their desired outcomes.

Post-session care is equally important, and the book outlines steps for immediate aftercare, relaxation techniques, and progress tracking. It also addresses common aftereffects and adjustments based on personal feedback.

Troubleshooting common issues is a key feature, offering solutions for scenarios such as not experiencing tremors or managing discomfort. It provides strategies for emotional releases and guidance on seeking professional support if needed.

The integration of TRE into daily life is explored, showing how to incorporate the practice into a regular routine, combine it with other healing methods, and use it for stress management. The book encourages readers to build a long-term practice plan and involves family and friends in their healing journey.

For those looking to advance their practice, the book delves into more sophisticated techniques, including adaptations for specific issues, advanced breathing methods, and continuing education resources, ensuring that readers can deepen their TRE practice and maximize its benefits.

Introduction to TRE

What TRE Is and Its Origins

Tension and Trauma Releasing Exercises (TRE) is a therapeutic method designed to help individuals release deep-seated stress and tension from their bodies. Developed by Dr. David Berceli, TRE focuses on the body's natural ability to heal itself through a series of simple exercises. Dr. Berceli created TRE after observing that the body naturally shakes or tremors in response to stress or trauma. His research into the physiological effects of these tremors led to the development of this technique, which aims to help individuals manage stress and trauma by harnessing the body's own mechanisms for healing.

Basic Principles of TRE

TRE is based on the principle that the body stores stress and trauma in its muscles and tissues. When the body experiences a traumatic event, it often enters a state of heightened tension, which can become chronic if not properly addressed. TRE consists of a series of exercises designed to induce a natural tremoring response in the body. This tremoring, or shaking, is believed to help release the accumulated stress and tension from the muscles. The exercises are simple and can be adjusted to suit individual needs, making TRE accessible to a wide range of people.

Benefits for Mental and Physical Health

TRE offers a variety of benefits for both mental and physical health. Physically, it helps to release muscle tension, reduce pain, and improve overall flexibility. Mentally, TRE can lead to reduced anxiety, improved sleep quality, and a greater sense of emotional well-being. By allowing the body to release built-up stress and trauma, TRE can also enhance resilience and improve overall mood. Many individuals report feeling more relaxed and centered after practicing TRE regularly, making it a valuable tool for managing stress and promoting mental health.

Common Misconceptions

Despite its benefits, TRE is sometimes misunderstood. One common misconception is that TRE is only for individuals who have experienced severe trauma. In reality, TRE can be beneficial for anyone looking to manage stress or improve overall well-being. Another misconception is that the tremoring response is a sign of a problem or that it should be suppressed. In fact, the tremoring is a natural and healthy response that helps the body release tension. TRE is also not a replacement for other forms of therapy but can be used in conjunction with them to enhance overall therapeutic outcomes.

How to Get Started

Getting started with TRE is straightforward and involves several key steps. First, it's important to find a qualified TRE provider or instructor who can guide you through the exercises and ensure you are practicing them correctly. Begin with a few basic exercises, gradually increasing their complexity as you become more comfortable. It's essential to listen to your body and proceed at your own pace. TRE can be practiced alone or in a group setting, depending on your preference. Regular practice is key to experiencing the full benefits of TRE, so setting aside dedicated time each week for the exercises will help you build and maintain progress.

CHAPTER ONE

THE SCIENCE BEHIND TRE

Tension and Trauma Releasing Exercises (TRE) are designed to help the body release deep-seated stress and trauma through the natural mechanism of tremors. These exercises leverage the body's inherent ability to shake off stress, a response observed in many animals. The science behind TRE revolves around the understanding of how our body processes and releases stored stress and trauma. By engaging in specific exercises, individuals trigger a series of involuntary muscle contractions that initiate a tremor response. This tremor mechanism is believed to help the body reset its stress response system and promote a state of relaxation and healing.

TRE is grounded in the concept that our muscles can hold onto stress and trauma long after the initial event. When we experience stress, our bodies go into a state of heightened alert, and muscles become tense. Over time, this tension can become chronic and difficult to release. TRE provides a way to stimulate the body's natural tremor response to help release this stored tension, enabling the body to return to a more balanced state. This approach is rooted in the principles of neurophysiology and bodywork, offering a practical method for managing stress and promoting emotional and physical well-being.

How TRE Affects The Nervous System

TRE affects the nervous system by targeting the autonomic nervous system, which controls involuntary bodily functions such as heart rate, digestion, and respiratory rate.

The autonomic nervous system is divided into the sympathetic nervous system (responsible for the fight-or-flight response) and the parasympathetic nervous system (responsible for rest and digestion).

TRE exercises stimulate the parasympathetic nervous system, helping to counteract the chronic activation of the sympathetic nervous system caused by stress.

During TRE, the tremor response helps to activate the parasympathetic nervous system, promoting a state of relaxation and reducing the overall stress response.

This shift from sympathetic to parasympathetic dominance allows the body to release tension and restore balance. As the tremors facilitate the release of stored stress, individuals often report a sense of calm and improved emotional regulation. This process helps to reset the body's stress response system, leading to enhanced overall well-being and resilience.

The Role Of Tremors In Healing

Tremors play a crucial role in the healing process facilitated by TRE. These involuntary muscle contractions, or tremors, are a natural response of the body to stress and trauma. When the body experiences stress, muscles can become tense and tight, holding onto this tension long after the stressor has been removed. Tremors help to release this stored tension by inducing a rhythmic shaking that targets the deep muscle layers and connective tissues.

The tremor response is thought to be a way for the body to reset its stress response system and promote relaxation. As the tremors occur, they stimulate the nervous system to release endorphins and other neurochemicals that aid in stress relief and emotional healing. This process helps to break the cycle of chronic tension and allows the body to recover from stress more effectively. By integrating tremors into the healing process, TRE provides a practical method for releasing built-up stress and promoting overall well-being.

Neurogenic Tremors Explained

Neurogenic tremors are tremors that originate from the nervous system and are often experienced as a response to stress or trauma. Unlike voluntary tremors, which are consciously controlled, neurogenic tremors are involuntary and arise from the body's natural stress response mechanisms.

These tremors occur when the nervous system is activated in response to stress or trauma, leading to a shaking or vibrating sensation in the muscles.

Neurogenic tremors are thought to be a natural way for the body to release accumulated stress and restore balance.

They are believed to help reset the autonomic nervous system, promoting a shift from the stress-induced sympathetic nervous system to the calming parasympathetic nervous system. This process aids in reducing muscle tension, improving emotional regulation, and facilitating overall healing.

By understanding neurogenic tremors, individuals can better appreciate how TRE harnesses this natural response to support stress relief and emotional well-being.

The Impact Of Stress On The Body

Stress has a profound impact on the body, influencing both physical and emotional health. When we experience stress, our bodies undergo a series of physiological changes designed to prepare us for a fight-or-flight response. This includes the release of stress hormones such as cortisol and adrenaline, which increase heart rate, blood pressure, and muscle tension. While these responses are helpful in the short term, chronic stress can lead to a range of health issues.

Long-term stress can result in persistent muscle tension, weakened immune function, digestive problems, and emotional disturbances such as anxiety and depression. The body's stress response system can become overloaded, leading to a state of constant alertness and fatigue. TRE addresses these issues by providing a method to release built-up tension and promote relaxation. By engaging in TRE, individuals can help mitigate the negative effects of stress and support their body's natural healing processes.

Research Findings On TRE's Effectiveness

Research on the effectiveness of TRE has demonstrated its potential benefits for stress reduction and trauma healing.

Studies have shown that TRE can significantly reduce symptoms of stress and anxiety by activating the body's natural tremor response. This process helps to release stored tension and promote relaxation, leading to improved emotional well-being.

Research also indicates that TRE can be effective in managing trauma and post-traumatic stress disorder (PTSD). By facilitating the release of deep-seated tension, TRE helps individuals process and recover from traumatic experiences. Clinical trials and anecdotal evidence suggest that regular practice of TRE can lead to long-term improvements in mental health and stress management.

Overall, TRE is supported by a growing body of research highlighting its effectiveness in promoting relaxation, reducing stress, and aiding in trauma recovery. As more studies are conducted, the understanding of TRE's benefits continues to evolve, providing valuable insights into its role in enhancing overall well-being.

CHAPTER TWO

SAFETY CONSIDERATIONS

When practicing Tension and Trauma Releasing Exercises (TRE), it's crucial to prioritize safety to ensure a beneficial and risk-free experience. Safety considerations revolve around understanding your body's limits, the environment in which you practice, and being aware of any pre-existing conditions that might affect your ability to perform TRE exercises.

Environment: Choose a safe, quiet, and comfortable space for your practice. Ensure the area is free from obstacles that could cause injury if you move around or lose balance. Using a yoga mat or a soft surface can provide additional comfort and support.

Physical Preparation: It's important to be well-hydrated and avoid eating a large meal right before practicing TRE. Wear comfortable clothing that allows for free movement and breathing.

Mindfulness: Pay close attention to your body's responses during exercises. Listen to your body's signals and be prepared to stop if you feel any pain or extreme discomfort. TRE is meant to release tension and trauma gently, so pushing beyond your limits can be counterproductive.

Who Should Practice Tre

TRE can be beneficial for many individuals, but it's especially valuable for those dealing with stress, anxiety, trauma, or chronic tension. Here are some guidelines on who should consider incorporating TRE into their wellness routine:

Stress and Anxiety: Those experiencing high levels of stress or anxiety may find TRE helpful in reducing physical tension and promoting relaxation.

The exercises are designed to trigger the body's natural stress-reducing mechanisms, helping to ease both physical and emotional stress.

Trauma Survivors: Individuals who have experienced trauma, whether it be emotional or physical, can benefit from TRE as it assists in processing and releasing stored tension.

It's advisable to work with a trained therapist when dealing with severe trauma to ensure a safe and supportive environment.

Chronic Pain Sufferers: People with chronic pain or muscle tension conditions may also find TRE useful. The exercises can help release muscle tightness and improve overall mobility.

General Wellness: Anyone interested in maintaining overall well-being and reducing stress might incorporate TRE into their routine as a preventative measure.

Potential Risks And Contraindications

Although TRE is generally safe for most people, there are certain risks and contraindications to be aware of.

Understanding these can help prevent potential issues and ensure that the practice remains beneficial.

Medical Conditions: Individuals with certain medical conditions, such as severe cardiovascular issues, significant joint problems, or recent surgeries, should consult with a healthcare provider before starting TRE. These conditions might require specific modifications or alternative approaches.

Pregnancy: Pregnant individuals should be cautious when practicing TRE. It's important to consult with a healthcare provider to determine if TRE is appropriate and to receive guidance on safe practices during pregnancy.

Mental Health Conditions: Those with severe mental health conditions, such as untreated PTSD or severe depression, should approach TRE with care.

Working with a mental health professional can help determine if TRE is suitable and ensure it is practiced safely.

How To Identify If TRE Is Right For You

Determining if TRE is right for you involves self-assessment and sometimes professional consultation. Here are steps to help you decide:

Self-Assessment: Reflect on your physical and emotional state. Are you dealing with chronic stress, muscle tension, or trauma? TRE can be beneficial if these issues align with your current needs. Evaluate how open you are to exploring new methods of stress relief and self-care.

Consultation: Speak with a healthcare provider or a TRE practitioner to discuss your specific situation.

They can help assess whether TRE aligns with your needs and offer guidance on how to start safely.

Trial and Observation: Start with a few introductory sessions of TRE to gauge how your body responds. Pay attention to how you feel both during and after the exercises.

If you experience positive changes and feel comfortable, TRE might be a good fit for you.

Safety Guidelines And Best Practices

Following safety guidelines and best practices will ensure a positive TRE experience and minimize any risks. Here's how to practice TRE safely:

Warm-Up: Begin with gentle warm-up exercises to prepare your body for TRE. This can include light stretching or mobility exercises to increase circulation and ease into the practice.

Start Slowly: Begin with shorter sessions and gradually increase the duration as you become more comfortable. It's important not to rush the process or overexert yourself.

Stay Grounded: Focus on maintaining a grounded and stable posture throughout the exercises. If you're practicing on the floor, ensure that you have adequate support and stability.

Hydrate and Rest: Drink plenty of water before and after your session to stay hydrated. Allow your body adequate time to rest and recover between sessions.

Seek Guidance: If you're unsure about any aspect of TRE or experience any issues, consult with a qualified TRE practitioner for guidance and adjustments to your practice.

What To Do If You Experience Discomfort

Experiencing discomfort during TRE can happen, especially if your body is new to the exercises. Here's how to manage and address discomfort:

Stop and Assess: If you feel significant discomfort or pain, stop the exercise immediately. Assess the type and intensity of the discomfort to determine if it's something that can be adjusted or if it requires further attention.

Modify the Exercise: Sometimes, discomfort can be alleviated by modifying the exercise. Adjust your position or technique to see if it helps reduce the discomfort.

Use Support: Utilize props such as cushions or yoga blocks to provide additional support and comfort during the exercises.

Consult a Professional: If discomfort persists or you're unsure about the cause, consult with a TRE practitioner or healthcare provider. They can offer advice on how to adjust your practice or determine if TRE is appropriate for you.

Rest and Recovery: Allow time for your body to rest and recover if you experience discomfort. Ensure you're not pushing beyond your limits and give yourself time to adjust to the exercises gradually.

CHAPTER THREE

PREPARING FOR THE

Creating A Practice Space

Creating a dedicated space for TRE (Tension & Trauma Releasing Exercises) is essential for an effective practice.

Ideally, your space should be quiet, private, and free from distractions. Choose a room or corner where you feel comfortable and relaxed. It should have enough room for you to lie down and move freely.

If possible, use soft lighting to create a calming atmosphere. You might want to add a few personal touches, such as calming colors or soothing decorations, to make the space inviting and conducive to relaxation.

Required Equipment And Attire

TRE doesn't require much equipment, making it accessible and easy to start. At a minimum, you'll need a comfortable mat or blanket to lie on.

This provides cushioning and support during the exercises. Some practitioners also use a bolster or cushion to support their back or legs, but this is optional.

Wear comfortable, loose-fitting clothing that allows for easy movement and doesn't restrict your body.

Avoid tight or restrictive clothes that might interfere with the exercises. Comfortable socks or being barefoot is generally preferred for better grip and relaxation.

Setting Up Your Practice Area

To set up your practice area, start by laying down your mat or blanket on a flat surface. Ensure that the space is clear of any obstacles or sharp objects that could potentially cause injury.

Arrange any additional props, like bolsters or cushions, within easy reach. Create a serene environment by adjusting the lighting and adding elements that help you feel at ease, such as calming music or essential oils.

If you prefer, you can also include a chair or small table to keep any notes or instructions handy. Make sure the area remains uncluttered to maintain a peaceful and focused practice.

Mental And Emotional Preparation

Before beginning TRE, take a moment to mentally and emotionally prepare yourself. This involves setting aside any stress or worries from your day.

Spend a few minutes in mindfulness or deep breathing exercises to center yourself. Acknowledge any emotions or physical sensations you may be experiencing, and remind yourself that TRE is a safe space to explore these feelings.

Embrace an attitude of curiosity and openness towards your body's responses. This mental preparation helps in creating a positive mindset, which enhances the effectiveness of the exercises.

How To Set Realistic Goals

Setting realistic goals for your TRE practice involves understanding what you hope to achieve and breaking it down into manageable steps. Start by identifying your primary objectives, such as reducing stress or releasing specific tension. Set small, achievable milestones to track your progress.

For example, you might aim to practice TRE for 10 minutes each day or complete a specific exercise routine.

Adjust your goals as needed based on how your body responds and how comfortable you feel with the exercises. Celebrate your progress and remain flexible, allowing your practice to evolve over time.

CHAPTER FOUR

THE TRE PRACTICE

Basic Exercises And Techniques

TRE, or Trauma Release Exercises, is a simple yet effective method designed to help release stress and tension held in the body.

The practice consists of a series of exercises that induce a natural tremor response, which helps to release deep-seated muscular tension. The core exercises involve a combination of stretching and shaking movements that encourage the body to process and release stored stress.

The foundational exercises in TRE are primarily designed to target the major muscle groups that often hold tension, such as the legs, back, and hips.

These exercises are straightforward, making them accessible for beginners and adaptable for those with varying levels of fitness.

How To Perform Each Exercise

Basic Leg Exercises: Start by lying on your back with your knees bent and feet flat on the floor.

Gently lift one leg at a time, and hold the position for a few seconds before switching legs. This movement helps to activate the muscles in your legs and lower back, setting the stage for the tremor response.

Hip Bridge: From the same starting position, lift your hips off the ground while keeping your shoulders and feet grounded. Hold this position for a few seconds, then lower your hips back down.

This exercise helps to strengthen and relax the muscles in your hips and lower back.

Back Stretch: While lying on your back, bring your knees to your chest and gently rock side to side. This motion helps to release tension in the lower back and hips.

Shaking Exercises: Stand with your feet shoulder-width apart and gently bounce on your heels. Allow your legs and arms to shake naturally. This shaking movement helps to stimulate the tremor response, promoting the release of stress.

Integrating Breathing Techniques

Breathing plays a crucial role in the effectiveness of TRE. Proper breathing techniques enhance the release of tension and support the tremor response. Begin by focusing on deep, diaphragmatic breaths. Inhale slowly through your nose, allowing your abdomen to expand, then exhale slowly through your mouth.

Incorporate breathing into your exercises by synchronizing your breaths with the movements. For instance, inhale as you lift your leg or hips, and exhale as you lower them. This practice helps to deepen the relaxation response and makes the tremors more effective.

Duration And Frequency Of Exercises

To achieve the best results, aim to practice TRE exercises regularly. Start with short sessions of about 10-15 minutes, 2-3 times a week. As you become more familiar with the exercises and your body adapts, you can gradually increase the duration to 20-30 minutes per session.

Consistency is key. Practicing TRE regularly helps to build resilience against stress and maintains the benefits of the tremor response. Adjust the frequency based on your individual needs and how your body responds to the exercises.

Common Adjustments For Different Needs

TRE can be adapted to accommodate various needs and fitness levels. If you have specific physical limitations or injuries, consider modifying the exercises to reduce strain.

For example, if you experience discomfort during the hip bridge exercise, you can perform a modified version by keeping your hips closer to the ground.

For those with limited mobility, focus on gentle, seated versions of the exercises. You can perform the leg exercises while seated in a chair, and use a wall or chair for support during the shaking exercises.

Adjust the intensity of the tremor response by varying the speed and amplitude of your movements. If you find the tremors too intense, slow down your shaking or reduce the range of motion.

By making these adjustments, TRE can be tailored to fit individual needs, ensuring that the practice remains accessible and beneficial for everyone.

CHAPTER FIVE

POST-SESSION CARE

What To Do Immediately After A Session

After completing a TRE (Tension and Trauma Release Exercises) session, it's essential to take some time to properly care for yourself to maximize the benefits and ensure a smooth recovery.

Begin by gently reorienting yourself to your surroundings. Take a few moments to sit quietly, breathe deeply, and allow your body to transition back from the exercise state. This calm period helps your nervous system shift back into a state of balance and readiness for daily activities.

Hydrate well by drinking water. TRE can be intense, and staying hydrated supports muscle recovery and overall well-being. If you've experienced any intense shaking or muscle activity, light stretching can help to ease any residual tension. Avoid jumping into strenuous activities immediately; instead, give yourself at least 30 minutes to an hour of rest before resuming your regular routine.

Post-Exercise Relaxation Techniques

To enhance the benefits of your TRE session, engage in relaxation techniques that promote recovery and relaxation. Progressive muscle relaxation is an excellent method to follow. Focus on tightening and then relaxing different muscle groups throughout your body. This practice helps in reducing any residual tension from the session and supports overall relaxation.

Mindfulness meditation is another valuable technique. Spend a few minutes sitting in a comfortable position, focusing on your breath, and observing any physical sensations or thoughts without judgment. This practice can help center your mind and further calm your body after TRE.

Consider taking a warm bath with Epsom salts to soothe any muscle soreness and promote relaxation. A warm bath can be particularly beneficial if you feel any lingering tension or tightness in your muscles.

How To Track And Record Your Progress

Tracking and recording your progress after TRE sessions is crucial for understanding how the exercises are affecting your body and mind. Start by maintaining a simple journal or digital record where you can note down the date, duration, and intensity of each session.

Include any observations about how you felt before, during, and after the session.

In your journal, document any changes in your physical or emotional state. For instance, note improvements in flexibility, reduction in muscle tension, or changes in mood.

Recording these details can help you identify patterns and make adjustments to your routine as needed.

You might also use a tracking app designed for fitness or wellness to monitor your progress. Many apps allow you to log various metrics, set goals, and review your progress over time, providing a comprehensive view of your TRE journey.

Common Aftereffects And How To Address Them

It's not uncommon to experience some aftereffects following a TRE session. These can include mild muscle soreness, fatigue, or emotional releases such as tears or mood swings. These responses are usually temporary and part of the body's natural healing process.

For muscle soreness, gentle stretching and hydration can be helpful. If soreness persists, applying a warm compress or engaging in light physical activity such as walking can alleviate discomfort.

If you encounter emotional releases, it's important to approach them with compassion and patience. Allow yourself time to process these emotions and consider speaking with a therapist or counselor if you need additional support. Journaling your feelings can also provide clarity and help in managing emotional responses.

Adjusting Your Routine Based On Feedback

Listening to your body and adjusting your TRE routine based on feedback is key to maximizing its benefits and ensuring long-term success. After each session, reflect on how your body responded and any changes in your overall well-being.

If you notice any areas of discomfort or unusual reactions, it may be necessary to modify your approach.

For example, if you experience excessive soreness or fatigue, you might need to reduce the intensity or frequency of your sessions.

On the other hand, if you find certain exercises particularly beneficial, you may choose to incorporate them more regularly into your routine.

Regularly review your progress notes and adjust your TRE routine based on your observations.

This iterative process ensures that your practice remains effective and aligned with your evolving needs and goals.

CHAPTER SIX

TROUBLESHOOTING COMMON ISSUES

What If You Don't Experience Tremors?

In TRE (Tension & Trauma Release Exercises), tremors are a common and often expected response, but not everyone experiences them. If you find that you're not shaking, it doesn't mean the exercises aren't working. First, ensure that you are following the exercises correctly and that your body is sufficiently relaxed. Sometimes, it takes time for your body to initiate the tremors, especially if you're new to TRE.

Consider checking your technique. Make sure you're in a comfortable position and allowing your body to relax completely. You might need to adjust the intensity or duration of your practice. If you're still not experiencing tremors, it may be helpful to review the exercises with a TRE practitioner who can provide personalized guidance.

Managing Discomfort During Practice

Experiencing discomfort during TRE practice is not uncommon, but it's important to manage it effectively to ensure a positive experience. If you feel discomfort, first assess whether it's due to improper technique or a physical limitation. Check your alignment and the surface you're working on. A supportive mat or cushion can often alleviate pressure.

Make sure you're not pushing yourself too hard. TRE should be practiced gently, allowing your body to adjust and respond at its own pace. If discomfort persists, consider taking breaks or modifying the exercises to better suit your comfort level. It's essential to listen to your body and avoid any movements that cause pain.

Dealing With Emotional Releases

TRE can sometimes trigger emotional releases, which are a natural part of the healing process. These releases can manifest as crying, laughter, or other emotional responses. It's crucial to acknowledge and accept these feelings as part of your body's way of processing stored tension.

Create a safe and supportive environment for yourself during practice. If you experience an emotional release, allow yourself to fully experience it without judgment. It may also be helpful to discuss your experiences with a trained TRE practitioner or therapist who can provide support and guidance through the process.

Adjusting Exercises For Different Levels

TRE exercises can be adapted to accommodate different skill levels and physical conditions. If you're a beginner or have specific physical limitations, start with simpler exercises and gradually progress as you become more comfortable. Focus on finding a level of intensity that feels manageable and beneficial for you.

For more advanced practitioners or those looking to deepen their practice, incorporating variations and additional exercises can be beneficial. Listen to your body and adjust the exercises based on how you're feeling. Working with a TRE practitioner can help tailor the exercises to fit your individual needs and goals.

Seeking Professional Guidance

If you encounter persistent issues or need additional support, seeking professional guidance can be invaluable. TRE practitioners are trained to help individuals navigate challenges and optimize their practice. They can provide personalized feedback, adjust exercises to better suit your needs, and offer strategies to address any difficulties you might be facing.

Consider reaching out to a certified TRE provider if you need assistance with technique, managing emotional releases, or adjusting exercises.

Their expertise can help you get the most out of your TRE practice and support your overall healing journey.

CHAPTER SEVEN

INTEGRATING TRE INTO DAILY LIFE

Integrating TRE (Tension and Trauma Releasing Exercises) into your daily life can significantly enhance your well-being and overall quality of life.

By making TRE a regular part of your routine, you can better manage stress, release tension, and promote emotional healing. Here's how to effectively incorporate TRE into your daily activities:

Incorporating TRE Into Your Daily Routine

To seamlessly integrate TRE into your daily routine, start by setting aside a specific time each day for your practice. Consistency is key to reaping the full benefits of TRE.

Choose a time that works best for you, whether it's in the morning to start your day on a positive note or in the evening to unwind and relax before bed.

Begin with short, manageable sessions, especially if you are new to TRE. Even just 5-10 minutes a day can be effective.

As you become more comfortable with the exercises, you can gradually increase the duration.

Creating a dedicated space in your home for TRE can also help reinforce the habit. Make sure this space is quiet, comfortable, and free from distractions.

Combining TRE With Other Healing Practices

TRE can be a powerful complement to other healing practices. Combining TRE with practices such as yoga, meditation, or mindfulness can amplify its benefits. For example, you might start your day with a short meditation session, followed by TRE exercises to release any accumulated tension. Yoga can also be an excellent addition, as it helps to enhance flexibility and promote overall relaxation, which can further support the effectiveness of TRE.

Consider integrating TRE into your existing wellness routine. If you practice mindfulness or relaxation techniques, use TRE as a way to deepen these practices. `

For instance, after a yoga session, perform TRE exercises to release any remaining tension in your muscles. This combination can lead to a more holistic approach to stress management and emotional healing.

Using TRE For Stress Management

TRE is particularly effective for managing stress. The exercises are designed to help your body release built-up tension and trauma, which can be a significant source of stress. To use TRE for stress management, identify the times when you feel most stressed or anxious and incorporate TRE exercises during those periods.

It can be helpful to combine TRE with stress-reducing techniques like deep breathing exercises. For instance, practice deep breathing before starting your TRE session to calm your mind and prepare your body for the release of tension.

This can enhance the overall effectiveness of the exercises and help you feel more relaxed and centered.

Creating A Long-Term Practice Plan

A long-term practice plan for TRE ensures that you maintain consistency and continue to benefit from the exercises over time. Start by setting realistic goals for your practice.

Determine how often you want to perform TRE and the duration of each session. Setting specific, achievable goals can help you stay motivated and track your progress.

Consider keeping a journal to record your experiences with TRE. Note any changes in your stress levels, physical sensations, or emotional state.

This can provide valuable insights into how TRE is impacting your life and help you adjust your practice plan as needed.

To keep your practice engaging, vary your TRE sessions by trying different exercises or incorporating new techniques.

Regularly revisiting your goals and progress can help you stay focused and committed to your long-term practice plan.

Encouraging Family And Friends To Join

Encouraging family and friends to join you in your TRE practice can enhance the experience and provide additional support.

Share the benefits of TRE with them and invite them to participate in a session. This can be particularly effective if you have a supportive community around you, as practicing together can strengthen relationships and create a shared commitment to well-being.

Offer to demonstrate the exercises and explain how TRE has positively impacted your life. Hosting group sessions or workshops can be a fun and interactive way to introduce others to TRE.

By creating a supportive environment and engaging others in the practice, you can help them experience the benefits of TRE and foster a collective approach to healing and stress management.

CHAPTER EIGHT

ADVANCED TRE TECHNIQUES

Exploring Deeper Techniques

Trauma Release Exercises (TRE) can be tailored beyond the basic practices to address more complex issues. Advanced TRE techniques involve incorporating more nuanced movements and mindfulness strategies to enhance the release of deep-seated trauma. One advanced method is using variations in body position to increase the intensity and focus of the tremors. For example, practitioners might use a combination of seated, lying, and standing positions to stimulate different muscle groups and release tension from various areas of the body.

Another advanced technique includes combining TRE with guided visualizations. By engaging in targeted imagery while performing exercises, you can deepen your awareness of internal sensations and emotional responses. This approach helps in addressing underlying psychological and emotional trauma that may not be fully accessed through physical exercise alone.

Adapting TRE For Specific Issues

TRE can be customized to address specific physical or emotional issues. For instance, if you are dealing with chronic back pain, you can modify the exercises to focus more on the back muscles and surrounding areas. This might involve adjusting the frequency and intensity of the tremor response in exercises like the "shaking" movement to target the lower back specifically.

For individuals with anxiety or stress-related disorders, TRE can be adapted to include calming techniques, such as slow, controlled breathing or mindfulness practices. This adaptation helps in not only releasing physical tension but also managing emotional responses. By integrating relaxation techniques with TRE, you can create a more holistic approach to managing and alleviating stress.

Combining TRE With Other Therapies

Integrating TRE with other therapeutic modalities can enhance overall effectiveness. Combining TRE with practices like yoga, acupuncture, or massage therapy can provide a comprehensive approach to trauma and stress relief. For instance, practicing yoga before or after TRE can help align the body and enhance the tremor response, while massage therapy can target areas of chronic tension that TRE may not fully address.

Another beneficial combination is TRE with cognitive-behavioral therapy (CBT). While TRE works on the physical release of trauma, CBT can address the cognitive and emotional aspects. This integrated approach allows for a more rounded healing process, addressing both the body and mind.

Advanced Breathing And Relaxation Methods

Advanced breathing techniques play a crucial role in enhancing the effectiveness of TRE. Techniques such as diaphragmatic breathing or alternate nostril breathing can help regulate the nervous system and facilitate a more profound tremor response. Practitioners can integrate these techniques before starting TRE to prepare the body for optimal release.

Relaxation methods, including progressive muscle relaxation or guided imagery, can further support the TRE process. By learning to relax deeply before and during TRE exercises, you can facilitate a smoother and more effective release of tension. This combination not only enhances the physical benefits of TRE but also supports emotional and mental relaxation.

Continuing Education And Resources

Ongoing education and access to resources are essential for mastering advanced TRE techniques. Workshops and advanced training sessions can provide deeper insights into the methodology and offer practical tips for applying these techniques in various scenarios. Engaging with online communities and forums dedicated to TRE can also provide valuable support and shared experiences.

Additionally, reading books and research papers on TRE can help in staying updated with the latest developments and methodologies. Resources such as instructional videos and professional guidance from certified TRE practitioners can further support your learning and application of advanced TRE techniques.